Contents

INTRODUCTION 3
    History and development 4
    Mechanism of action 7
    Uses and applications 11
Medical Uses of Mifepristone 15
    Abortion Pill Regimen 15
    Emergency Contraception 18
    Treatment of Cushing's Syndrome 22
    Potential future applications 26
Safety and Efficacy 31
    Side Effects and Risks: 35
    Effectiveness Rates: 37
Legal and Ethical Considerations 40
    Impact on reproductive rights 44
Patient Counseling and Education 49
    Managing expectations and concerns 54
Practical Guidelines for Healthcare Providers 59
    Follow-up Care and Monitoring: 64
    Handling Complications and Emergencies: 67
Comparative Analysis 72
    Comparison with Other Abortion Methods: 72
    Comparing Different Mifepristone Regimens: 75

Global Perspectives 80
    Availability and Accessibility: 80
    Cultural and Societal Attitudes:..81
    Challenges in Implementation: 82
Research and Innovation 86
    Ongoing Research Areas: 86
    Potential Developments in Mifepristone Usage: 88
CONCLUSION...91

INTRODUCTION

Mifepristone, often known as the "abortion pill" or RU-486, is a medication that plays a pivotal role in medical abortion procedures. It belongs to a class of drugs called antiprogestogens and works by blocking the hormone progesterone, which is crucial for maintaining pregnancy. This disruption causes the lining of the uterus to break down, leading to the detachment of the embryo or fetus.

Introduced in the 1980s, mifepristone has revolutionized reproductive healthcare by offering a non-surgical alternative for terminating early pregnancies. Beyond abortion, it is also used in combination with misoprostol for emergency contraception and in the treatment of conditions like Cushing's syndrome. Despite its widespread use, mifepristone remains a subject of debate and controversy in many regions due to ethical, legal, and societal concerns surrounding abortion and reproductive rights.

In medical settings, mifepristone is administered under strict guidelines to ensure safety and effectiveness. It requires informed consent and careful monitoring to manage potential side effects and ensure the patient's well-being. Ongoing research continues to explore new applications and formulations of mifepristone, promising further advancements in reproductive healthcare.

History and development

The history and development of mifepristone is a fascinating journey marked by scientific breakthroughs and societal implications. Here's an overview:

1. Discovery and Development:

   - 1960s-1970s: Mifepristone (originally known as RU-38486) was developed by a team of researchers led by Drs. Georges Teutsch and Étienne-Émile Baulieu at the French pharmaceutical company Roussel-Uclaf. The research aimed to create a compound that could act as a contraceptive by blocking progesterone receptors.

- 1980s: After extensive testing, mifepristone was identified as an antiprogestin, meaning it could block the effects of progesterone in the body. This property made it suitable not only for contraceptive purposes but also for inducing abortion in early pregnancy.

2. Introduction as an Abortifacient:

- 1988: Mifepristone received approval in France for use as an abortifacient, marking a significant milestone in reproductive healthcare. This approval was based on clinical trials demonstrating its effectiveness in safely inducing abortion when followed by misoprostol.

3. Global Impact and Controversies:

- 1990s-2000s: The introduction of mifepristone sparked debates worldwide regarding abortion rights, ethical considerations, and legal frameworks. Its availability and acceptance varied widely between countries, influenced by cultural, religious, and political factors.

- United States: Mifepristone faced regulatory challenges and political scrutiny. It was approved by the FDA in 2000 under the brand name Mifeprex, but with strict prescribing and dispensing regulations, often referred to as REMS (Risk Evaluation and Mitigation Strategy) requirements.

4. Expanded Uses and Research:

- Beyond Abortion: Mifepristone's utility expanded beyond abortion to include treatment for conditions such as Cushing's syndrome (a hormonal disorder) and research into its potential in cancer therapy due to its anti-progestational effects.

5. Future Directions:

   - Ongoing research continues to explore new applications and formulations of mifepristone, aiming to improve safety, efficacy, and accessibility. Potential future uses include management of endometriosis and other gynecological disorders.

In summary, the history and development of mifepristone reflect its evolution from a scientific discovery to a pivotal tool in reproductive healthcare, influencing medical practice, public policy, and societal attitudes towards abortion and contraception globally.

Mechanism of action

The mechanism of action of mifepristone revolves around its ability to interact with progesterone receptors in the body. Here's a detailed explanation:

1. Progesterone Receptors:

   - Progesterone is a hormone crucial for maintaining pregnancy by preparing the uterine lining for implantation of a fertilized egg and supporting early pregnancy. Progesterone exerts its effects by binding to specific receptors (progesterone receptors) located in the uterus and other tissues.

2. Antiprogestin Activity:

   - Mifepristone is classified as an antiprogestin because it competitively binds to these progesterone receptors with a higher affinity than progesterone itself. By binding to these receptors, mifepristone blocks the biological effects of progesterone.

3. Effects on the Uterus:

   - In the context of medical abortion:

- Early Pregnancy: Mifepristone is administered orally, typically in combination with misoprostol. In early pregnancy (up to 10 weeks gestation), mifepristone disrupts the action of progesterone in the uterus. This disruption leads to:

    - Softening and dilation of the cervix.

    - Thinning and breakdown of the uterine lining (endometrium), which reduces the ability to sustain the pregnancy.

    - Detachment of the embryo or fetus from the uterine wall, leading to its expulsion.

4. Synergistic Effect with Misoprostol:

    - After mifepristone treatment, misoprostol (a prostaglandin analogue) is typically administered to induce uterine contractions, facilitating the expulsion of the embryo or fetus and completion of the abortion process.

5. Other Uses:

   - Emergency Contraception: Mifepristone can also be used in higher doses as an emergency contraceptive if administered shortly after unprotected intercourse. Here, it prevents implantation of a fertilized egg by altering the uterine environment.

   - Medical Conditions: In conditions like Cushing's syndrome, mifepristone blocks the effects of cortisol (a hormone produced in excess in Cushing's syndrome) by antagonizing glucocorticoid receptors.

6. Safety and Monitoring:

   - Mifepristone's mechanism of action necessitates careful medical supervision to ensure appropriate dosing, timing, and management of potential side effects such as bleeding and cramping.

In conclusion, mifepristone's mechanism of action as an antiprogestin underlies its effectiveness in medical abortion, emergency contraception, and treatment of certain medical conditions. Understanding its interactions with progesterone receptors is crucial for optimizing its therapeutic use and safety.

Uses and applications

Mifepristone has several important uses and applications across reproductive health and beyond. Here's a detailed overview:

1. Medical Abortion:

   - Primary Use: Mifepristone is primarily used in combination with misoprostol for medical abortion up to 10 weeks of gestation. This regimen is highly effective and offers a non-surgical option for terminating early pregnancies.

   - Procedure: Mifepristone is administered orally to block progesterone receptors, leading to the breakdown of the uterine lining and detachment of the embryo or fetus. Misoprostol is then used to induce contractions and complete the abortion process.

2. Emergency Contraception:

   - Post-Coital Use: Mifepristone can be used in higher doses as emergency contraception if taken shortly after unprotected intercourse. It prevents implantation of a fertilized egg by altering the uterine environment, thereby acting as a contraceptive method.

3. Treatment of Cushing's Syndrome:

   - Anti-Glucocorticoid Activity: Mifepristone blocks the action of cortisol at the glucocorticoid receptors, making it useful in the treatment of Cushing's syndrome. This condition is characterized by excessive levels of cortisol in the body, leading to various health issues.

4. Research and Potential Future Uses:

- Endometriosis: There is ongoing research into the use of mifepristone for the management of endometriosis, a condition where tissue similar to the lining of the uterus grows outside the uterus.

- Fibroids: Some studies suggest mifepristone may be beneficial in treating uterine fibroids by reducing their size and symptoms.

- Cancer Therapy: Due to its anti-progestational effects, mifepristone is being explored in research for its potential role in cancer therapy, particularly in hormone-dependent cancers.

5. Experimental Uses:

- Psychiatric Disorders: There is experimental research exploring mifepristone's potential in treating psychiatric disorders such as depression, bipolar disorder, and psychotic disorders, although its use in these areas is still investigational.

6. Off-Label Uses:

   - In some cases, mifepristone may be used off-label for conditions not approved by regulatory agencies, based on clinical judgment and research findings.

7. Ethical and Legal Considerations:

   - The use of mifepristone in medical abortion remains a topic of ethical and legal debate in many countries, impacting its availability and accessibility.

In summary, mifepristone is a versatile medication with applications ranging from medical abortion and emergency contraception to the treatment of specific medical conditions like Cushing's syndrome. Ongoing research continues to explore its potential in various other areas of healthcare, promising further advancements in reproductive and general medicine.

Medical Uses of Mifepristone

Abortion Pill Regimen

Mifepristone, also known as the abortion pill or RU-486, is a key component in medical abortion, which provides a non-surgical option for terminating early pregnancies. Here's how mifepristone is used in this context:

1. Administration and Mechanism of Action:

   - Dosage: Mifepristone is typically administered orally in a clinic or healthcare setting.

   - Mechanism: It works by blocking the action of progesterone, a hormone necessary for maintaining pregnancy. Progesterone prepares the uterus for implantation and sustains the pregnancy by maintaining the uterine lining.

   - Effect: By blocking progesterone receptors, mifepristone causes the lining of the uterus to break down, preventing further development of the pregnancy.

2. Combination with Misoprostol:

   - Procedure: Mifepristone is often followed by a prostaglandin analog called misoprostol, which is usually taken buccally (placed in the cheek pouch) or vaginally 24-48 hours after mifepristone administration.

   - Role of Misoprostol: Misoprostol induces uterine contractions, leading to expulsion of the products of conception, including the embryo or fetus, and the uterine lining.

3. Effectiveness and Safety:

   - High Success Rate: The mifepristone-misoprostol regimen is highly effective, with success rates typically exceeding 95% when used within the recommended gestational age (up to 10 weeks of pregnancy).

   - Safety Profile: Medical abortion using mifepristone and misoprostol is generally considered safe when administered under medical supervision. Common side effects include cramping, bleeding, nausea, and diarrhea, which are managed with appropriate medical guidance.

4. Advantages:

   - Non-surgical Option: It offers an alternative to surgical abortion procedures, which some individuals may prefer due to personal, medical, or logistical reasons.

   - Privacy and Control: Medical abortion allows individuals to manage the process in the privacy of their home, following initial clinic visits for mifepristone administration and guidance.

5. Considerations and Counseling:

   - Informed Decision: Counseling and informed consent are crucial aspects of the medical abortion process. Healthcare providers discuss the procedure, potential side effects, expected outcomes, and follow-up care with patients.

- Follow-Up: Follow-up visits or consultations ensure that the abortion is complete and that the patient's health and well-being are monitored.

In summary, mifepristone plays a pivotal role in medical abortion by disrupting progesterone activity and initiating the process of pregnancy termination. Its use in combination with misoprostol offers a safe and effective non-surgical option for early pregnancy termination, providing individuals with reproductive choice and autonomy.

Emergency Contraception

1. Mechanism of Action:

- Mifepristone, when used as emergency contraception, prevents pregnancy primarily by inhibiting the action of progesterone. Progesterone is essential for maintaining the uterine lining and preparing it for implantation of a fertilized egg. By blocking progesterone receptors, mifepristone alters the endometrium, making it less receptive to implantation.

2. Timing and Administration:

- Post-Coital Use: Mifepristone is taken orally as a single dose as soon as possible after unprotected intercourse, ideally within 72 hours (3 days) but potentially up to 120 hours (5 days) after.

- Dosage: The typical dose for emergency contraception with mifepristone is higher than that used for medical abortion, often around 10 to 50 mg, depending on the protocol used.

3. Effectiveness:

- Efficacy: Mifepristone used as emergency contraception has been shown to reduce the risk of pregnancy when taken within the specified timeframe.

However, its effectiveness may vary compared to other emergency contraception methods like levonorgestrel or ulipristal acetate.

- Factors Affecting Effectiveness: The effectiveness of emergency contraception with mifepristone may depend on various factors, including the timing of administration relative to ovulation and individual factors affecting hormone levels.

4. Safety and Side Effects:

- Safety Profile: Mifepristone used for emergency contraception is generally considered safe, but like any medication, it can have side effects such as nausea, abdominal pain, fatigue, and changes in menstrual bleeding.

- Monitoring: As with any form of emergency contraception, individuals using mifepristone should be monitored for any adverse effects and provided with appropriate medical guidance.

5. Availability and Use:

   - Regulatory Considerations: Availability of mifepristone for emergency contraception may vary by region and country, as regulatory approvals and guidelines can influence its accessibility.

   - Consultation and Counseling: Individuals considering mifepristone for emergency contraception should consult healthcare providers for guidance on proper use, potential side effects, and follow-up care.

In summary, while less commonly used than other emergency contraception methods like levonorgestrel or ulipristal acetate, mifepristone offers an alternative for preventing pregnancy after unprotected intercourse. Its mechanism of action involves blocking progesterone receptors to alter the uterine environment, reducing the likelihood of implantation. As with any medication, individuals should consult healthcare providers to discuss the most appropriate emergency contraception method based on individual circumstances and medical advice.

Mifepristone also finds application in the treatment of Cushing's syndrome, a condition caused by prolonged exposure to high levels of cortisol. Here's an overview of how mifepristone is utilized in this context:

Treatment of Cushing's Syndrome

1. Mechanism of Action:

   - Anti-Glucocorticoid Activity: Mifepristone acts as an antagonist at the glucocorticoid receptor sites, blocking the effects of cortisol. This action reduces the binding of cortisol to its receptors, thereby mitigating its metabolic, cardiovascular, and psychiatric effects.

2. Indications and Use:

   - Cushing's Syndrome: This condition results from either an overproduction of cortisol by the adrenal glands (endogenous Cushing's syndrome) or prolonged use of corticosteroid medications (exogenous Cushing's syndrome). Mifepristone is primarily used in cases of endogenous Cushing's syndrome where surgical intervention is not feasible or has not been successful in controlling the symptoms.

3. Clinical Benefits:

 - Symptom Control: Mifepristone helps alleviate the symptoms associated with Cushing's syndrome, such as weight gain, central obesity (fat accumulation in the trunk and face), hypertension, glucose intolerance, and psychological disturbances.

 - Quality of Life: By reducing the effects of excess cortisol, mifepristone can improve patients' quality of life and reduce the complications associated with Cushing's syndrome.

4. Dosage and Administration:

- Dosage: Mifepristone is typically administered orally, with the dosage tailored to individual patient needs and response.

- Monitoring: Regular monitoring of cortisol levels, metabolic parameters (such as glucose tolerance), and potential side effects is essential during treatment with mifepristone.

5. Safety and Side Effects:

- Side Effects: Common side effects of mifepristone in the treatment of Cushing's syndrome may include fatigue, nausea, headache, dizziness, and alterations in potassium and blood pressure levels.

- Adverse Events: Serious adverse events, such as adrenal insufficiency or liver enzyme elevations, although rare, require close monitoring and management.

6. Considerations:

- Patient Selection: Proper patient selection, including consideration of the underlying cause and severity of Cushing's syndrome, is crucial for the appropriate use of mifepristone.

- Multidisciplinary Care: Treatment of Cushing's syndrome often involves collaboration among endocrinologists, surgeons, and other healthcare providers to optimize patient outcomes and manage potential complications.

In summary, mifepristone's ability to antagonize glucocorticoid receptors makes it a valuable option for managing symptoms associated with Cushing's syndrome, particularly in cases where surgical intervention is not suitable or sufficient. Its use requires careful monitoring and management to ensure safety and efficacy in improving patient outcomes and quality of life.

Potential future applications

Looking ahead, mifepristone holds promise for several potential future applications beyond its current uses. Here are some areas where ongoing research and exploration are focused:

1. Endometriosis:

   - Mifepristone's ability to modulate hormone receptors makes it a candidate for treating endometriosis, a condition where tissue similar to the lining of the uterus grows outside the uterus. Research suggests it may help reduce symptoms such as pelvic pain and menstrual irregularities associated with endometriosis.

2. Uterine Fibroids:

   - Studies have explored mifepristone's potential in treating uterine fibroids, non-cancerous growths in the uterus. It may help shrink fibroids and alleviate symptoms such as heavy menstrual bleeding and pelvic pressure.

3. Breast Cancer:

   - Mifepristone's anti-progestational effects have sparked interest in its potential role in treating hormone-sensitive breast cancers. Research is ongoing to determine its efficacy and safety in combination with other therapies.

4. Psychiatric Disorders:

   - There is ongoing research into mifepristone's potential therapeutic benefits in psychiatric disorders such as depression, bipolar disorder, and psychotic disorders. Its ability to modulate stress hormone receptors (including glucocorticoid receptors) may offer new avenues for treatment.

5. Cancer Therapy:

   - Beyond breast cancer, mifepristone is being investigated in preclinical and clinical studies for its potential in other types of cancer, including ovarian cancer and certain types of meningiomas (brain tumors).

6. Autoimmune Disorders:

   - Some research suggests that mifepristone may have immunomodulatory effects that could be beneficial in autoimmune disorders. Further studies are needed to explore its potential applications in conditions like rheumatoid arthritis and lupus.

7. Male Contraception:

   - Mifepristone's ability to block progesterone and other hormonal pathways has raised interest in its potential as a component of male contraceptive methods. Research is ongoing to develop safe and effective hormonal contraceptives for men.

8. Other Gynecological Conditions:

   - There is ongoing exploration into mifepristone's potential in treating other gynecological conditions, such as polycystic ovary syndrome (PCOS), where hormonal imbalances play a significant role.

9. Anti-inflammatory Effects:

   - Mifepristone's anti-inflammatory properties may be beneficial in conditions where inflammation plays a central role, such as certain types of arthritis and inflammatory bowel disease (IBD).

10. Neurological Disorders:

   - Preliminary research suggests that mifepristone may have neuroprotective effects and could potentially be useful in neurodegenerative disorders like Alzheimer's disease and Parkinson's disease.

In conclusion, while mifepristone is currently established in medical abortion, emergency contraception, and the treatment of Cushing's syndrome, ongoing research continues to explore its potential in diverse areas of healthcare. Future applications of mifepristone hold promise for expanding its therapeutic utility across various medical conditions and improving patient outcomes.

Safety and Efficacy

In discussing the safety and efficacy of mifepristone, particularly through clinical trials and research studies, several key aspects come to light:

1. Clinical Trials Overview:

- Early Development: Mifepristone underwent rigorous clinical trials during its development phase in the late 20th century. These trials focused initially on its effectiveness in terminating early pregnancies and its safety profile.

- Abortion Regimen: Clinical trials evaluated the combination of mifepristone with misoprostol for medical abortion, assessing factors such as efficacy rates, completeness of abortion, and side effects.

- Dose Optimization: Studies aimed to determine the optimal dosage of mifepristone for various indications, balancing effectiveness with safety considerations.

2. Safety Profile:

- Adverse Events: Clinical trials have documented common adverse events associated with mifepristone use, including nausea, vomiting, abdominal pain, diarrhea, and dizziness. Serious complications, such as heavy bleeding requiring intervention, are rare but monitored closely.

- Long-term Safety: Long-term safety data have been collected to assess any potential risks associated with mifepristone use, particularly in cases where it may be used off-label or in higher doses for medical conditions like Cushing's syndrome.

3. Efficacy in Different Applications:

- Medical Abortion: Clinical trials have consistently shown high efficacy rates for the mifepristone-misoprostol regimen in terminating early pregnancies, typically exceeding 95% when used within recommended gestational limits.

- Emergency Contraception: Studies have evaluated mifepristone's effectiveness as emergency contraception when taken shortly after unprotected intercourse, demonstrating its ability to reduce the risk of pregnancy when administered within the appropriate timeframe.

- Cushing's Syndrome: Trials and observational studies have demonstrated mifepristone's efficacy in controlling symptoms of Cushing's syndrome, including improvements in weight, blood pressure, and glucose metabolism markers.

4. Comparative Studies:

- Versus Surgical Methods: Comparative trials have assessed mifepristone's effectiveness and patient preferences compared to surgical abortion methods, highlighting its non-invasive nature and acceptability.

- Emergency Contraception: Research has compared mifepristone with other emergency contraception methods like levonorgestrel and ulipristal acetate, examining efficacy rates and side effect profiles.

5. Ethical and Regulatory Considerations:

- Informed Consent: Ethical guidelines require informed consent processes in clinical trials involving mifepristone, ensuring patients understand the risks, benefits, and alternatives.

- Regulatory Oversight: Regulatory agencies monitor ongoing research and clinical use of mifepristone to ensure adherence to safety standards and to update prescribing information based on emerging data.

In conclusion, clinical trials and research studies have been instrumental in establishing the safety, efficacy, and appropriate use of mifepristone across its approved indications. Ongoing research continues to refine its applications and monitor long-term outcomes, contributing to evidence-based healthcare practices and patient safety.

Side Effects and Risks:
1. Common Side Effects:

   - Gastrointestinal: Nausea, vomiting, diarrhea, and abdominal pain are among the most commonly reported side effects of mifepristone. These symptoms are usually mild to moderate and typically resolve without intervention.

- Vaginal Bleeding: Heavy or prolonged vaginal bleeding is expected after taking mifepristone, especially when followed by misoprostol for medical abortion. This bleeding is part of the natural process of expelling the uterine contents.

- Other: Dizziness, fatigue, headache, and fever can also occur but are less common.

2. Serious Risks:

- Incomplete Abortion: In a small percentage of cases, medical abortion with mifepristone and misoprostol may result in incomplete abortion, requiring additional intervention or surgical evacuation.

- Infection: Although rare, there is a risk of pelvic infection following medical abortion, which requires prompt medical attention if symptoms such as fever, pelvic pain, or abnormal vaginal discharge occur.

- Allergic Reactions: Allergic reactions to mifepristone are rare but can include rash, itching, swelling, or difficulty breathing.

3. Long-term Safety:

- Data Limitations: Long-term safety data for mifepristone, particularly in off-label uses or higher doses for conditions like Cushing's syndrome, are still evolving. Monitoring for potential risks such as adrenal insufficiency and liver enzyme elevations is essential in these cases.

Effectiveness Rates:
1. Medical Abortion:

- High Success Rates: When used within the recommended gestational age (up to 10 weeks of pregnancy), the mifepristone-misoprostol regimen is highly effective, with success rates typically exceeding

95%. Effectiveness may vary slightly based on factors such as gestational age and individual response.

  - Completion Rates: Studies indicate that approximately 98-99% of women successfully have a complete abortion with the mifepristone-misoprostol regimen.

2. Emergency Contraception:

  - Reduced Pregnancy Risk: Mifepristone used as emergency contraception within 72 hours (up to 120 hours in some protocols) of unprotected intercourse has been shown to reduce the risk of pregnancy. Effectiveness rates can vary, but studies suggest it may be comparable to other emergency contraception methods.

3. Treatment of Cushing's Syndrome:

  - Symptomatic Improvement: Clinical trials have demonstrated that mifepristone effectively reduces symptoms associated with Cushing's syndrome, such as weight gain, hypertension, and glucose intolerance. Improvement rates vary, but a significant proportion of patients experience substantial relief.

In summary, while mifepristone is generally well-tolerated and highly effective in its approved uses, it is important for healthcare providers and patients to be aware of potential side effects, risks, and effectiveness rates associated with its various applications. Adherence to prescribed protocols, informed consent, and careful monitoring contribute to optimizing safety and outcomes in clinical practice.

Legal and Ethical Considerations

Legal and ethical considerations surrounding mifepristone encompass a complex landscape influenced by cultural, religious, political, and healthcare perspectives. Here's an overview of key aspects:

Legal Considerations:

1. Regulatory Approval:

   - Global Variability: The legal status of mifepristone varies widely across countries and regions. Some countries have approved its use for medical abortion and other indicated uses, while others have restrictions or outright bans.

   - Regulatory Agencies: Approval and regulation often involve health authorities or regulatory bodies that assess safety, efficacy, and appropriate use based on clinical data and public health considerations.

2. Access and Availability:

- Healthcare Systems: Accessibility to mifepristone can be influenced by healthcare infrastructure, policies, and provider training. Availability may vary between urban and rural areas and may be restricted by legal barriers or logistical challenges.

- Reproductive Rights: Legal frameworks may impact access to mifepristone as part of broader reproductive rights debates, including access to abortion services and emergency contraception.

Ethical Considerations:

1. Reproductive Autonomy:

- Patient Rights: Ethical discussions often center on the right of individuals to make informed decisions about their reproductive health, including access to safe and legal abortion services.

- Informed Consent: Ensuring informed consent processes, including comprehensive information about risks, benefits, and alternatives, is crucial in ethical healthcare delivery involving mifepristone.

2. Healthcare Provider Autonomy:

   - Conscientious Objection: Healthcare providers may have conscientious objections to prescribing or administering mifepristone based on religious, moral, or ethical beliefs. Legal frameworks in some jurisdictions accommodate such objections while ensuring access to care.

3. Public Health Impact:

   - Public Policy: Ethical considerations extend to public health policies that aim to balance individual rights with population health outcomes, including reducing unsafe abortions and improving maternal health.

4. Stigma and Discrimination:

- Social Attitudes: Stigma and discrimination related to abortion and contraception can influence legal and ethical debates surrounding mifepristone, impacting access and public discourse.

5. Advocacy and Human Rights:

- Advocacy Efforts: Organizations and advocates work to protect and promote reproductive rights, including access to mifepristone and comprehensive reproductive healthcare services.

- Human Rights Framework: Ethical arguments often invoke human rights principles, emphasizing dignity, equality, and non-discrimination in healthcare access and decision-making.

In conclusion, legal and ethical considerations surrounding mifepristone reflect diverse societal perspectives and ongoing debates about reproductive rights, healthcare access, and ethical healthcare practices. These considerations shape policies, practices, and public discourse, impacting the availability and use of mifepristone in healthcare systems worldwide.

Impact on reproductive rights

Mifepristone has a significant impact on reproductive rights, influencing debates and policies related to abortion access, emergency contraception, and broader reproductive healthcare. Here's an exploration of its impact:

1. Access to Safe Abortion:

   - Alternative to Surgical Abortion: Mifepristone, used in combination with misoprostol, provides a non-surgical option for terminating early pregnancies. Its availability expands options for individuals seeking abortion services, particularly in regions where access to surgical procedures may be limited or restricted.

   - Legal and Regulatory Challenges: Legal frameworks governing mifepristone's use vary globally, impacting accessibility and affordability. Advocates for reproductive rights argue for policies that ensure safe and legal access to mifepristone and comprehensive abortion care.

2. Emergency Contraception:

  - Preventing Unintended Pregnancies: Mifepristone's role as emergency contraception offers individuals a preventive option after unprotected intercourse. Its availability supports reproductive autonomy by allowing timely decision-making regarding pregnancy prevention.

  - Legal and Regulatory Barriers: Challenges in regulatory approval and availability of emergency contraception formulations containing mifepristone affect access and awareness, particularly in conservative or restrictive legal environments.

3. Autonomy and Informed Choice:

- Patient-Centered Care: Reproductive rights encompass the principle of autonomy, empowering individuals to make informed decisions about their reproductive health. Informed consent processes for mifepristone ensure that individuals receive comprehensive information about risks, benefits, and alternatives.

- Ethical Considerations: Ethical debates center on respecting individual choices and protecting healthcare provider autonomy while navigating conscientious objections and ensuring equitable access to reproductive healthcare services.

4. Public Health and Social Justice:

- Reducing Unsafe Abortions: Access to mifepristone contributes to public health goals by reducing reliance on unsafe abortion methods, which pose significant health risks to individuals.

- Addressing Inequities: Socioeconomic factors, geographic disparities, and legal restrictions impact access to mifepristone and reproductive healthcare services, highlighting social justice implications in ensuring equitable access for all individuals, regardless of background or circumstance.

5. Legal and Policy Advocacy:

  - Advocacy Efforts: Organizations and activists advocate for policies that protect and promote reproductive rights, including access to mifepristone and comprehensive reproductive healthcare services.

  - Human Rights Framework: Reproductive rights are framed within human rights principles, emphasizing dignity, equality, non-discrimination, and the right to health in advocating for policies that support access to mifepristone and reproductive healthcare.

In summary, mifepristone's impact on reproductive rights extends beyond its clinical applications, shaping legal frameworks, public health policies, and ethical discourse surrounding abortion access, emergency contraception, and reproductive healthcare. Its availability and regulatory status influence individuals' ability to exercise informed choice and access safe and timely reproductive healthcare services worldwide.

Patient Counseling and Education

Patient counseling and education regarding mifepristone are crucial aspects of ensuring safe and informed healthcare decisions. Here's a comprehensive overview:

1. Counseling Before Administration:

- Medical Indications: Healthcare providers explain the specific medical indications for mifepristone, such as medical abortion, emergency contraception, or treatment of conditions like Cushing's syndrome.

- Procedure Explanation: Patients receive detailed information about the mifepristone regimen, including dosing, timing, and the potential need for additional medications like misoprostol in the case of medical abortion.

- Alternative Options: Providers discuss alternative treatment options available for the patient's specific medical condition, outlining their respective benefits, risks, and efficacy.

2. Informed Consent:

- Understanding Risks and Benefits: Patients are informed about the potential risks and side effects associated with mifepristone, such as nausea, abdominal pain, vaginal bleeding, and less common but serious complications like incomplete abortion or infection.

- Efficacy and Expected Outcomes: Counseling includes a discussion on the effectiveness rates of mifepristone for its intended use, ensuring that patients have realistic expectations about treatment outcomes.

- Follow-Up Care: Patients are advised on the importance of follow-up appointments or monitoring to assess treatment effectiveness, manage side effects, and address any concerns or complications that may arise.

3. Safety Precautions and Considerations:

- Contraindications and Precautions: Providers review medical conditions, medications, or allergies that may contraindicate the use of mifepristone or require special precautions.

- Emergency Contact Information: Patients receive instructions on when and how to seek immediate medical attention in case of severe symptoms or complications, such as excessive bleeding, severe abdominal pain, or signs of infection.

4. Emotional and Psychological Support:

- Counseling Support: Recognizing the emotional aspects of reproductive healthcare decisions, healthcare providers offer supportive counseling and resources to address patients' emotional needs before and after mifepristone administration.

- Respecting Patient Choices: Providers respect patients' autonomy and decisions regarding their reproductive health, offering non-judgmental support and ensuring that patients feel empowered throughout the process.

5. Access and Practical Guidance:

- Accessibility: Patients receive information about where to obtain mifepristone and related medications, as well as any logistical considerations such as travel to a healthcare facility or local regulations affecting access.

- Instructions for Use: Clear instructions are provided on how to take mifepristone as prescribed, including timing, administration route, and any necessary precautions or dietary restrictions.

6. Continued Support and Follow-Up:

- Monitoring and Follow-Up: Providers emphasize the importance of scheduled follow-up visits to monitor treatment effectiveness, manage any ongoing symptoms, and address any questions or concerns that arise post-treatment.

- Long-Term Considerations: For conditions requiring long-term mifepristone use, such as Cushing's syndrome, patients receive education on ongoing monitoring, potential adjustments in treatment, and long-term health implications.

In summary, comprehensive patient counseling and education on mifepristone ensure that individuals make informed decisions, understand treatment expectations, and receive the necessary support throughout their healthcare journey. Effective communication and patient-centered care are essential in promoting safety, adherence to treatment protocols, and overall well-being.

Managing expectations and concerns

Managing expectations and addressing concerns are critical aspects of patient counseling and education regarding mifepristone. Here's how healthcare providers can effectively navigate these areas:

1. Managing Expectations:

- Treatment Outcomes: Provide clear and accurate information about the expected outcomes of mifepristone treatment based on the patient's specific indication (e.g., medical abortion, emergency contraception, or treatment of Cushing's syndrome).

- Effectiveness: Discuss the effectiveness rates of mifepristone for its intended use, ensuring that patients have realistic expectations about the likelihood of success and the potential need for additional interventions or follow-up care.

- Timeline: Explain the timeline for expected effects and recovery, including when symptoms such as bleeding or cramping may occur and how long they typically last.

2. Addressing Concerns:

- Side Effects and Risks: Educate patients about common side effects such as nausea, abdominal pain, and vaginal bleeding, as well as less common but serious risks like incomplete abortion or infection. Provide reassurance about the management of these symptoms and when to seek medical attention.

- Safety: Address concerns about the safety of mifepristone, emphasizing its approval by regulatory authorities and the extensive clinical research supporting its use in safe and effective healthcare practices.

- Alternative Options: Discuss alternative treatment options available for their medical condition, including their benefits, risks, and how they compare to mifepristone, respecting patient preferences and individual circumstances.

3. Providing Support:

- Emotional Support: Recognize the emotional aspects of reproductive healthcare decisions and provide empathetic support. Encourage open communication about feelings, concerns, and any anxieties related to the treatment process.

- Information Accessibility: Ensure patients have access to educational materials, resources, and contact information for further questions or support needs before, during, and after treatment.

4. Respecting Autonomy:

- Informed Decision-Making: Empower patients to make informed decisions about their reproductive health by providing comprehensive information, respecting their values and preferences, and involving them in shared decision-making processes.

- Cultural Sensitivity: Respect cultural beliefs and values that may influence patient perspectives on reproductive healthcare decisions, ensuring that counseling and support are culturally competent and respectful.

5. Follow-Up and Continued Care:

- Scheduled Visits: Emphasize the importance of scheduled follow-up visits to monitor treatment effectiveness, manage any ongoing symptoms or concerns, and adjust treatment plans as needed.

- Long-Term Management: For conditions requiring long-term mifepristone use, such as Cushing's syndrome, discuss long-term management strategies, including ongoing monitoring, potential side effects, and lifestyle considerations.

In summary, effective management of expectations and concerns involves providing clear, compassionate, and personalized counseling and education. By addressing these aspects proactively, healthcare providers can enhance patient understanding, confidence in treatment decisions, and overall satisfaction with their healthcare experience involving mifepristone.

Practical Guidelines for Healthcare Providers

1. Medical Abortion:

- Initial Assessment:

  - Confirm pregnancy through clinical history and testing.

  - Assess gestational age to ensure eligibility (typically up to 10 weeks gestation).

- Administration Protocol:

  - Administer mifepristone orally at a standard dose (usually 200 mg).

  - Provide instructions for subsequent administration of misoprostol (typically 24-48 hours later) to induce uterine contractions and complete abortion.

- Monitoring:

- Advise patients on expected symptoms (bleeding, cramping) and provide guidelines for managing discomfort.

- Schedule follow-up visit to confirm completion of abortion and assess any complications.

2. Emergency Contraception:

- Timing and Administration:

  - Offer mifepristone as emergency contraception within 72 hours (up to 120 hours in some protocols) of unprotected intercourse.

  - Administer a single oral dose (usually 50 mg).

- Follow-Up:

  - Discuss the need for ongoing contraception and provide options for long-term contraceptive methods.

- Educate on potential menstrual changes or side effects following administration.

3. Treatment of Cushing's Syndrome:

- Patient Selection:

  - Confirm diagnosis of Cushing's syndrome through clinical and laboratory evaluation.

  - Assess patient suitability for mifepristone therapy based on severity of symptoms and underlying health conditions.

- Administration Protocol:

  - Initiate therapy at a low dose (e.g., 300-600 mg/day) and titrate based on clinical response and tolerability.

  - Monitor adrenal function and metabolic parameters regularly to assess treatment efficacy and safety.

- Long-Term Management:

  - Plan for ongoing monitoring of symptoms, adrenal function tests, and potential adjustments in medication dosage.

  - Educate patients on the importance of adherence to treatment and regular follow-up visits.

4. General Administration Guidelines:

- Contraindications and Precautions:

  - Review contraindications (e.g., allergy to mifepristone, ectopic pregnancy) and precautions (e.g., concurrent use of certain medications) before administration.

  - Adjust dosage or consider alternative treatments as necessary based on individual patient factors.

- Documentation and Follow-Up:

- Document administration details, patient education, informed consent, and any adverse reactions.

- Schedule follow-up visits to assess treatment outcomes, manage side effects, and address patient concerns.

5. Legal and Ethical Considerations:

- Adherence to Regulations:

  - Familiarize yourself with local laws and regulations governing the use of mifepristone for medical abortion, emergency contraception, and off-label uses.

  - Ensure compliance with institutional policies and ethical guidelines related to reproductive healthcare.

- Informed Consent:

  - Provide comprehensive information on treatment options, risks, benefits, and alternatives to support informed decision-making by patients.

- Respect patient autonomy and preferences throughout the treatment process, including considerations of cultural and personal beliefs.

By adhering to these practical guidelines, healthcare providers can effectively manage the administration of mifepristone across its approved indications, ensuring safe and patient-centered care while promoting positive healthcare outcomes and patient satisfaction.

Certainly! Here are practical guidelines for healthcare providers regarding follow-up care, monitoring, handling complications, and emergencies related to mifepristone:

Follow-up Care and Monitoring:
1. Medical Abortion:

- Scheduled Follow-up Visit:

  - Schedule a follow-up visit approximately 7-14 days after mifepristone administration to assess completion of abortion and manage any residual products of conception if needed.

- Confirm absence of pregnancy through clinical evaluation, which may include pelvic examination, ultrasound, or laboratory tests.

- Symptom Management:

  - Educate patients on expected post-abortion symptoms (bleeding, cramping) and provide guidance on managing discomfort at home.

  - Advise on when to seek medical attention for concerning symptoms such as severe pain, heavy bleeding, or signs of infection.

2. Emergency Contraception:

- Follow-up Counseling:

- Discuss the importance of ongoing contraception and provide options for long-term contraceptive methods to prevent future unintended pregnancies.

  - Address any concerns or questions regarding menstrual changes or potential side effects following emergency contraception.

- Monitoring:

  - Recommend follow-up contact or visit as needed to assess patient satisfaction with emergency contraception and address any ongoing contraceptive needs or concerns.

3. Treatment of Cushing's Syndrome:

- Regular Monitoring:

  - Establish a schedule for ongoing monitoring of symptoms, adrenal function tests (e.g., cortisol levels), and metabolic parameters (e.g., glucose tolerance, lipid profile).

- Monitor for improvement in clinical symptoms such as weight gain, hypertension, and glucose intolerance, adjusting treatment as necessary.

- Long-term Management:

  - Plan for periodic follow-up visits to evaluate treatment efficacy, manage side effects, and assess patient adherence to therapy.

  - Educate patients on the importance of continued medication adherence and regular medical supervision for optimal management of Cushing's syndrome.

Handling Complications and Emergencies:
1. Medical Abortion:

- Recognizing Complications:

- Educate patients on warning signs of complications such as heavy bleeding, severe abdominal pain, fever, or signs of infection.

- Provide clear instructions on when to seek immediate medical attention, including after-hours or emergency contact information.

- Management of Incomplete Abortion:

  - Prepare to manage cases of incomplete abortion with additional medication (e.g., misoprostol) or surgical intervention (e.g., vacuum aspiration) as necessary.

  - Ensure access to appropriate medical facilities equipped to handle complications related to medical abortion.

2. Emergency Contraception:

- Side Effects Management:

- Address potential side effects of emergency contraception (e.g., nausea, headache) and provide supportive care recommendations.

- Monitor for any adverse reactions and offer reassurance regarding the transient nature of most side effects.

3. Treatment of Cushing's Syndrome:

- Managing Adverse Events:

- Monitor for potential adverse events associated with mifepristone therapy, such as adrenal insufficiency, hypokalemia, or liver enzyme abnormalities.

- Implement appropriate management strategies based on clinical presentation and laboratory findings.

- Emergency Preparedness:

- Educate patients on signs of adrenal crisis (e.g., severe fatigue, weakness, hypotension) and the need for prompt medical evaluation in case of acute symptoms.

  - Ensure patients have access to emergency medical services and clear instructions on when and how to seek urgent care.

Documentation and Communication:

- Record Keeping:

  - Maintain accurate documentation of follow-up visits, treatment outcomes, patient education, and any interventions or complications encountered.

  - Facilitate continuity of care by sharing relevant information with other healthcare providers involved in the patient's treatment.

- Patient Communication:

- Communicate openly and transparently with patients about follow-up care plans, monitoring schedules, and expectations for ongoing management.

- Encourage patients to ask questions, express concerns, and actively participate in decisions regarding their healthcare.

By following these guidelines, healthcare providers can ensure comprehensive follow-up care, effective monitoring, and prompt management of complications or emergencies related to mifepristone administration. This approach supports patient safety, enhances treatment outcomes, and promotes patient satisfaction and confidence in their healthcare experience.

Comparative Analysis

Let's delve into a comparative analysis of mifepristone with other abortion methods, as well as a comparison of different mifepristone regimens used for various medical indications:

Comparison with Other Abortion Methods:

1. Medical Abortion (Mifepristone + Misoprostol) vs. Surgical Abortion:

- Effectiveness:

  - Medical abortion with mifepristone and misoprostol is highly effective, with success rates typically exceeding 95% when used within the recommended gestational age (up to 10 weeks).

  - Surgical abortion, such as vacuum aspiration or dilation and evacuation (D&E), also has high success rates and may be preferred for later gestational ages or when medical abortion is contraindicated.

- Procedure:

  - Medical abortion involves a non-surgical approach using medications (mifepristone followed by misoprostol) to induce abortion and expel the pregnancy tissue.

  - Surgical abortion requires a procedure performed in a clinical setting by a trained healthcare provider to remove the pregnancy tissue from the uterus.

- Safety:

  - Both methods are generally safe when performed under appropriate medical supervision. Medical abortion carries risks of incomplete abortion or infection, while surgical abortion carries risks associated with anesthesia and procedural complications.

- Patient Preference:

- Patient preference may vary based on factors such as gestational age, personal comfort with medical procedures, access to healthcare facilities, and cultural or religious beliefs.

2. Medical Abortion (Mifepristone + Misoprostol) vs. Manual Vacuum Aspiration (MVA):

- Procedure:

  - MVA involves using a handheld device to manually suction out the pregnancy tissue from the uterus, often performed in early pregnancies (up to 10 weeks).

  - Medical abortion with mifepristone and misoprostol involves medication-induced expulsion of the pregnancy tissue at home or in a clinical setting.

- Effectiveness and Safety:

- Both methods are highly effective and safe when performed correctly by trained providers. MVA may offer quicker completion of the procedure compared to medical abortion, which may take several hours to days.

- Accessibility and Preference:

  - Medical abortion with mifepristone and misoprostol may be more accessible in settings where surgical facilities or anesthesia services are limited.

  - Patient preference may vary based on factors such as privacy, convenience, and individual healthcare needs.

Comparing Different Mifepristone Regimens:
1. Standard Medical Abortion Regimen (Mifepristone + Misoprostol):

- Dosage and Timing:

  - Mifepristone is typically administered orally at a dose of 200 mg, followed by misoprostol 24-48 hours later to induce uterine contractions and complete abortion.

- Effectiveness:

  - High success rates exceeding 95% for complete abortion within the recommended gestational age (up to 10 weeks), with most patients experiencing expulsion of pregnancy tissue within 24 hours of misoprostol administration.

- Safety Profile:

  - Common side effects include nausea, vomiting, abdominal pain, and vaginal bleeding. Serious complications such as incomplete abortion or infection are rare but possible.

2. Emergency Contraception Regimen:

- Dosage and Timing:

  - Mifepristone is administered as emergency contraception within 72 hours (up to 120 hours in some protocols) of unprotected intercourse, typically at a lower dose (e.g., 50 mg).

- Effectiveness:

  - Offers a preventive option to reduce the risk of pregnancy by preventing implantation of a fertilized egg. Effectiveness rates vary but may be comparable to other emergency contraception methods.

- Safety and Side Effects:

  - Generally well-tolerated with mild side effects such as nausea or headache. No long-term adverse effects on fertility or future pregnancies have been reported.

3. Treatment of Cushing's Syndrome:

- Dosage and Duration:

- Mifepristone is used at higher doses (e.g., 300-1200 mg/day) for the management of hypercortisolism in patients with Cushing's syndrome.

- Mechanism of Action:

  - Blocks the glucocorticoid receptor, reducing cortisol activity and alleviating symptoms such as weight gain, hypertension, and glucose intolerance.

- Effectiveness and Monitoring:

  - Efficacy varies among patients, requiring regular monitoring of clinical symptoms, adrenal function tests, and metabolic parameters to optimize treatment outcomes and manage potential side effects.

In summary, mifepristone offers a versatile option for medical abortion, emergency contraception, and the management of Cushing's syndrome, each with specific dosing regimens, effectiveness profiles, safety considerations, and patient preferences. Healthcare providers play a crucial role in educating patients, discussing treatment options, and ensuring personalized care based on individual medical needs and circumstances.

Global Perspectives

Availability and Accessibility:

1. Regional Disparities:

   - Developed Countries: Mifepristone is generally available and accessible in developed countries with established healthcare systems. It is often integrated into reproductive healthcare services and available in clinics, hospitals, and pharmacies.

   - Developing Countries: Accessibility varies widely. In some regions, mifepristone may be restricted or unavailable due to regulatory barriers, limited healthcare infrastructure, or cultural and political opposition to abortion.

2. Legal and Regulatory Landscape:

   - Legal Status: The legal status of mifepristone varies globally. It may be fully legalized, restricted to specific uses (e.g., medical abortion), or banned altogether in some countries.

- Regulatory Challenges: Regulatory approval processes, importation restrictions, and political dynamics influence availability and access, impacting healthcare provider training and public awareness.

3. Healthcare Infrastructure:

- Urban-Rural Disparities: Accessibility can be limited in rural or remote areas where healthcare facilities offering mifepristone may be scarce or non-existent.

- Health Worker Training: Adequate training of healthcare providers in mifepristone administration and management is essential but may be lacking in resource-constrained settings.

Cultural and Societal Attitudes:
1. Religious and Ethical Perspectives:

- Abortion Debate: Cultural and religious beliefs strongly influence societal attitudes toward abortion and, consequently, mifepristone use.

- Stigma and Discrimination: Stigma surrounding abortion and reproductive healthcare services may deter individuals from seeking mifepristone or other related services, impacting accessibility and healthcare seeking behavior.

2. Gender Norms and Rights:

- Women's Rights: Access to mifepristone intersects with broader issues of women's rights and reproductive autonomy. Societal attitudes toward gender roles and rights impact policy debates and implementation efforts.

- Informed Decision-Making: Cultural norms regarding family planning, contraception, and reproductive health literacy affect individuals' ability to make informed decisions about mifepristone use.

Challenges in Implementation:
1. Policy and Legal Barriers:

- Restrictive Legislation: Legal restrictions, including bans on mifepristone or stringent regulations, hinder access and implementation efforts.

- Policy Advocacy: Advocacy for policy reforms, based on evidence-based practices and human rights frameworks, is crucial to expanding access and reducing barriers.

2. Health System Integration:

- Healthcare Provider Training: Ensuring healthcare providers are trained in mifepristone administration, counseling, and management of complications is essential but may face challenges in resource-limited settings.

- Supply Chain Management: Ensuring reliable supply chains for mifepristone and related medications is critical for sustained availability and accessibility.

3. Public Awareness and Education:

- Stigma Reduction: Public education campaigns can help reduce stigma surrounding abortion and mifepristone use, promoting accurate information and destigmatizing reproductive healthcare services.

- Community Engagement: Engaging community leaders, religious institutions, and civil society organizations in discussions about reproductive health rights and mifepristone can foster supportive environments for implementation efforts.

Conclusion:

Global perspectives on mifepristone reflect a complex interplay of legal, cultural, societal, and health system factors. Addressing challenges in availability, accessibility, cultural attitudes, and implementation requires comprehensive strategies that prioritize human rights, evidence-based practices, and equitable healthcare access for all individuals, regardless of geographical location or socio-cultural context. Advocacy, policy reform, healthcare provider training, and public education are integral to advancing global reproductive health goals and ensuring the safe and effective use of mifepristone worldwide.

Research and Innovation

Ongoing Research Areas:

1. Expanded Indications:

   - Cancer Treatment: Research is exploring mifepristone's potential as an anti-cancer agent, particularly in hormone-sensitive cancers like breast and ovarian cancer.

   - Psychiatric Disorders: Studies are investigating mifepristone as a treatment for psychiatric conditions such as depression, bipolar disorder, and psychosis, targeting glucocorticoid receptor modulation.

2. Improving Treatment Protocols:

   - Dosing Regimens: Research aims to optimize mifepristone dosing for various indications, including medical abortion, emergency contraception, and Cushing's syndrome, to enhance efficacy and minimize side effects.

- Combination Therapies: Investigating combination therapies with mifepristone and other medications to improve treatment outcomes or mitigate adverse effects.

3. Mechanism of Action Studies:

- Molecular Pathways: Understanding the molecular mechanisms underlying mifepristone's actions beyond glucocorticoid receptor antagonism, including effects on progesterone and other receptor pathways.

- Impact on Cellular Processes: Research exploring mifepristone's effects on cellular signaling pathways, apoptosis, and gene expression in different disease models.

4. Long-Term Safety and Efficacy:

- Clinical Trials: Continued monitoring and evaluation of long-term safety profiles and efficacy outcomes in diverse patient populations, including reproductive-aged women and individuals with chronic conditions like Cushing's syndrome.

Potential Developments in Mifepristone Usage:
1. Precision Medicine Approaches:

   - Personalized Treatment: Advancing towards personalized medicine approaches based on genetic and biomarker profiles to tailor mifepristone therapy for individual patient needs.

   - Targeted Therapies: Developing targeted therapies using mifepristone for specific subtypes of diseases or conditions based on molecular characteristics.

2. Alternative Formulations:

   - Extended-Release Formulations: Developing extended-release formulations of mifepristone to prolong therapeutic effects and improve patient adherence, particularly in chronic disease management.

- Alternative Routes of Administration: Exploring alternative routes (e.g., transdermal, subcutaneous) for mifepristone administration to enhance convenience and patient comfort.

3. Emerging Technologies:

 - Nanotechnology: Investigating nanotechnology-based delivery systems for mifepristone to enhance drug delivery efficiency, bioavailability, and tissue targeting.

 - Gene Editing: Exploring potential applications of mifepristone in gene editing technologies, such as CRISPR-based therapies, to modulate gene expression in disease contexts.

4. Healthcare Innovation:

 - Telemedicine Integration: Integrating mifepristone administration and follow-up care into telemedicine platforms to improve accessibility and reach underserved populations.

  - Digital Health Tools: Utilizing digital health tools and mobile applications for patient education, adherence monitoring, and real-time support in mifepristone therapy management.

In conclusion, ongoing research in mifepristone spans various therapeutic areas and innovative approaches, aiming to expand its clinical utility, improve treatment outcomes, and address unmet medical needs. Continued advancements in understanding its mechanisms of action, exploring novel formulations, and leveraging emerging technologies hold promise for enhancing mifepristone's role in modern healthcare practices.

CONCLUSION

In conclusion, mifepristone stands as a versatile medication with significant implications across reproductive health, endocrinology, and potentially beyond. This comprehensive guide has explored various facets of mifepristone, highlighting its mechanisms of action, diverse medical applications, safety considerations, legal and ethical implications, patient counseling strategies, and global perspectives. Here are key takeaways:

1. Medical Applications: Mifepristone is primarily known for its role in medical abortion, emergency contraception, and the management of conditions like Cushing's syndrome. Its ability to selectively antagonize progesterone and glucocorticoid receptors makes it valuable in both reproductive health and endocrine disorders.

2. Safety and Efficacy: Understanding the safety profile and efficacy rates of mifepristone is crucial for healthcare providers and patients alike. While generally safe when administered under appropriate medical supervision, it does carry potential risks and requires careful monitoring.

3. Legal and Ethical Considerations: The availability and accessibility of mifepristone are influenced by legal frameworks, cultural attitudes toward abortion, and healthcare infrastructure. Advocacy for reproductive rights and evidence-based policymaking play pivotal roles in expanding access and ensuring safe usage.

4. Patient Counseling and Education: Effective patient counseling involves managing expectations, addressing concerns, and providing comprehensive information about mifepristone's benefits, risks, and alternatives. Respect for patient autonomy and cultural sensitivity are essential in facilitating informed decision-making.

5. Global Perspectives: Mifepristone's availability varies globally, reflecting diverse regulatory landscapes, cultural beliefs, and healthcare disparities. Overcoming challenges in implementation requires collaborative efforts to promote access, reduce stigma, and integrate reproductive healthcare into broader health systems.

6. Research and Innovation: Ongoing research aims to broaden mifepristone's therapeutic applications, refine treatment protocols, explore novel formulations, and advance personalized medicine approaches. Emerging technologies and scientific advancements hold promise for enhancing its efficacy and expanding its clinical utility.

In essence, mifepristone exemplifies the intersection of medical science, public health policy, and societal values. Its continued evolution and integration into healthcare practices depend on continuous research, advocacy for reproductive rights, and equitable access to safe and effective healthcare for all individuals worldwide.

www.ingramcontent.com/pod-product-compliance
Lightning Source LLC
Chambersburg PA
CBHW070344230526
45471CB00006B/2430